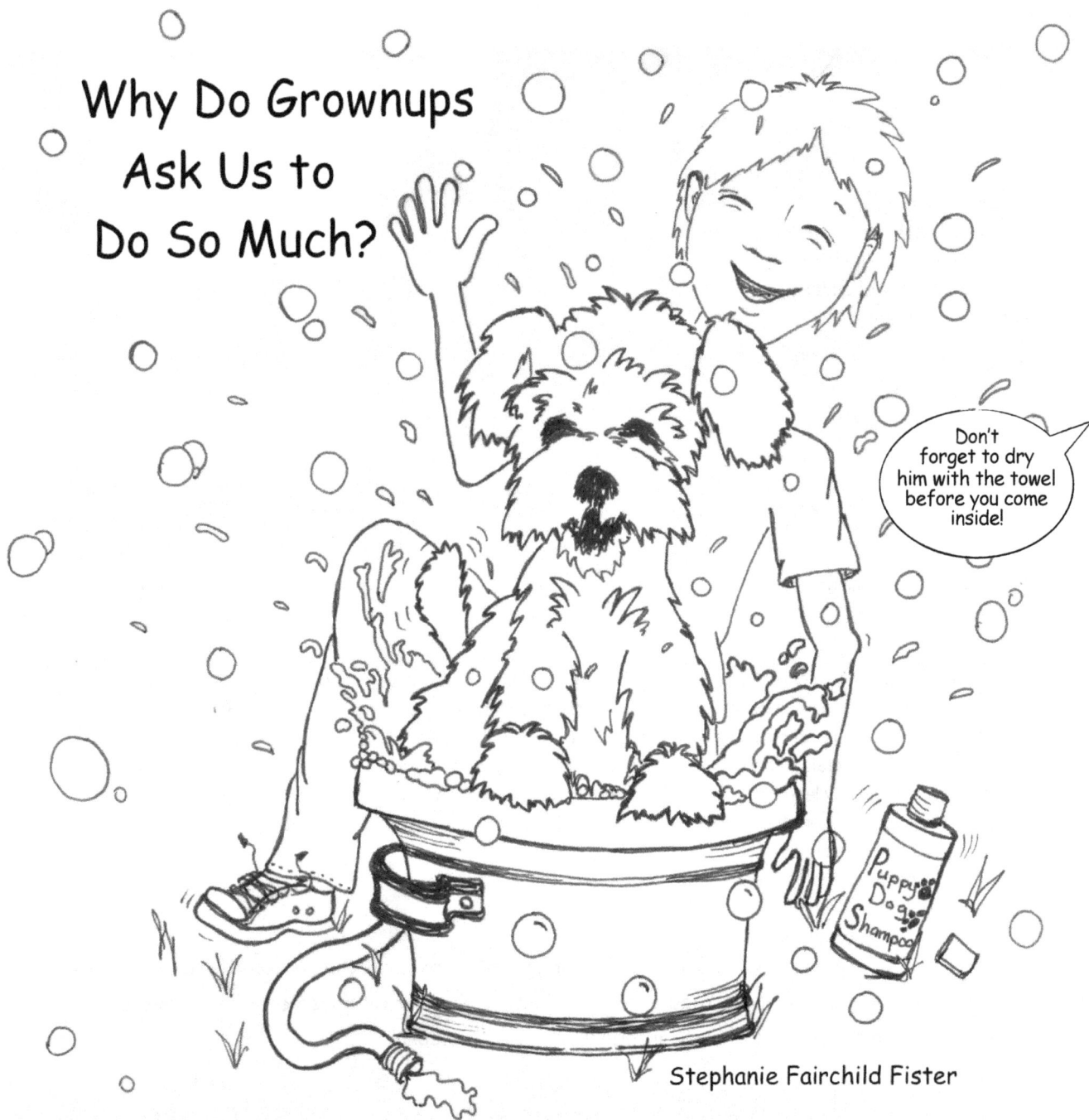

What's Best for Our Kids
   Publishing

For information: WhatsBestForOurKids.com

Whats Best for Our Kids™
and Whats Best for Our Kids ™
design logos are trademarks owned by
Whats Best for Our Kids™
Lexington, Kentucky. All rights reserved.

First printing: 2015

Library of Congress Cataloging-in-publication Data
Fister, Stephanie Fairchild
ISBN 978-0-9740064-0-8

Children want to have fun and be childlike while adults often ask them to sit, listen, write complete sentences, and solve long math problems over and over again. This book invites children to understand the answer to the big question of why the grownups in their lives ask them to stay inside and learn new lessons when the playground is calling their names. It explains how a balance of learning, wise choices, play, rest, and healthy food will help them get where they want to go in life. Teachers and parents can use this book as a curriculum for building healthy learning climates. Building a healthy learning climate must be exciting and fun in order to allow children to feel safe, comfortable, and motivated to pursue their potential as individuals and as a generation.

1. Juvenile Nonfiction: Careers
2. Juvenile Nonfiction: Family-Parents
3. Juvenile Nonfiction: General

Printed in the United States of America

The book Why Do Grown Ups Ask Us to Do So Much is printed with the font Dyslexie. These letters are designed to make reading faster, easier, and more enjoyable for all readers, especially those with dyslexia. For more information: Dyslexie.com

Dedicated to children of all ages

Time to wake up
and
get dressed by yourself,

and let's eat
a good breakfast together.

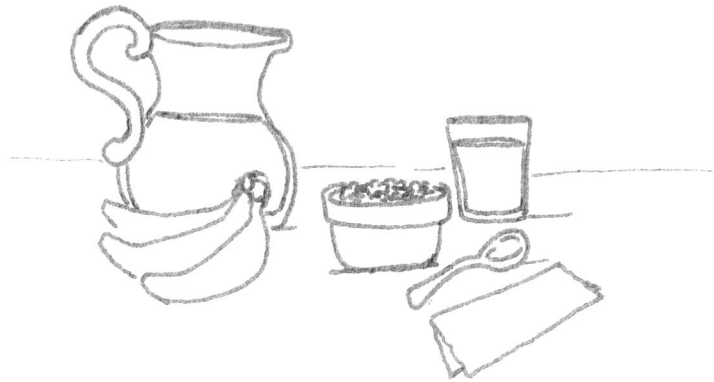

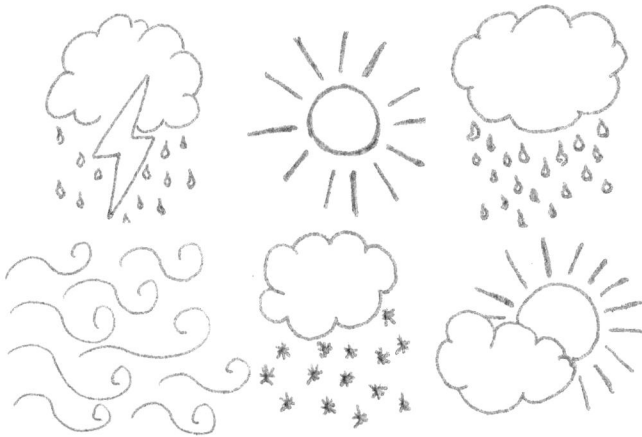

Laugh a little, make a plan,

and be sure to
check on the weather.

A jacket? A hat?
Which shoes will do?

A good start makes
the day better
all the way through!

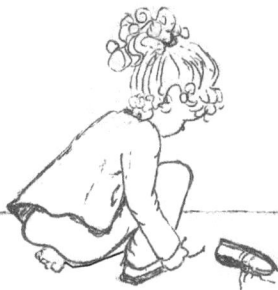

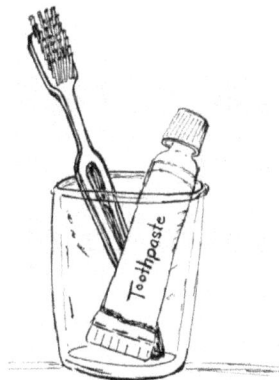

So don't forget to brush your teeth,
and wash your smiley face.

Oh my it's time for school, let's go!

We might
just have
to race!

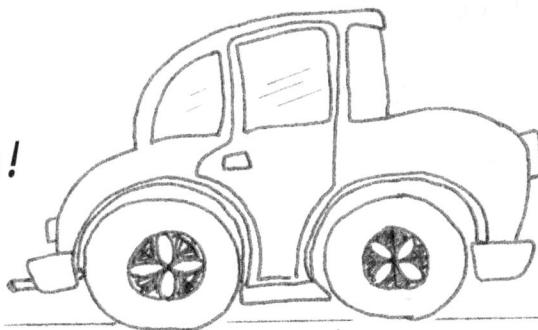

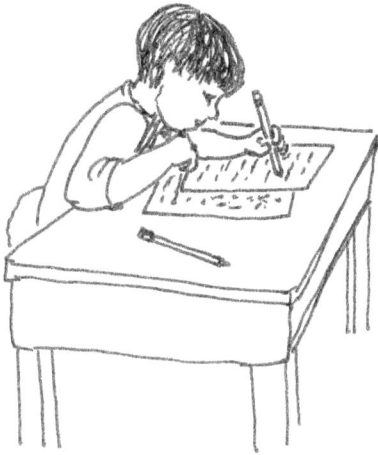

It's time to sit. Read a book.
Listen to this lesson well.

Solve this page of math problems,
here's twenty words to spell.

Now, let us sing
a song a while,
then run around
the gym
three times.

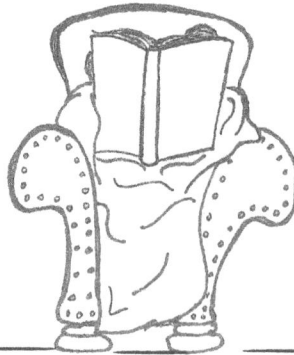

Home to play, eat,
and brush,
next read a book
like this one... that
rhymes!

Oh, how much grownups ask you to do,
and you always must do what they say.

Why can't you just go to the park,
and eat yummy cookies all day?

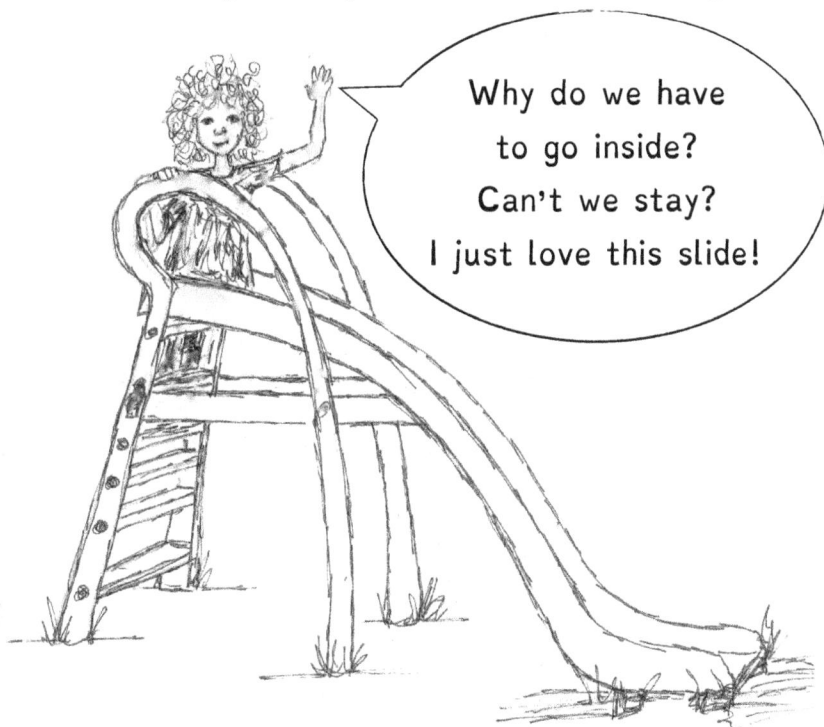

Why do we have
to go inside?
Can't we stay?
I just love this slide!

You see, we grownups were once kids too,
not such a long time ago,
and an answer to this question
we really want you to know!

So we're telling you why we ask so much
in every day of every season,
but first you must know this,
the things we ask fit into one of three big reasons.

Grownups ask what they ask,
not to bug you with a boring task,

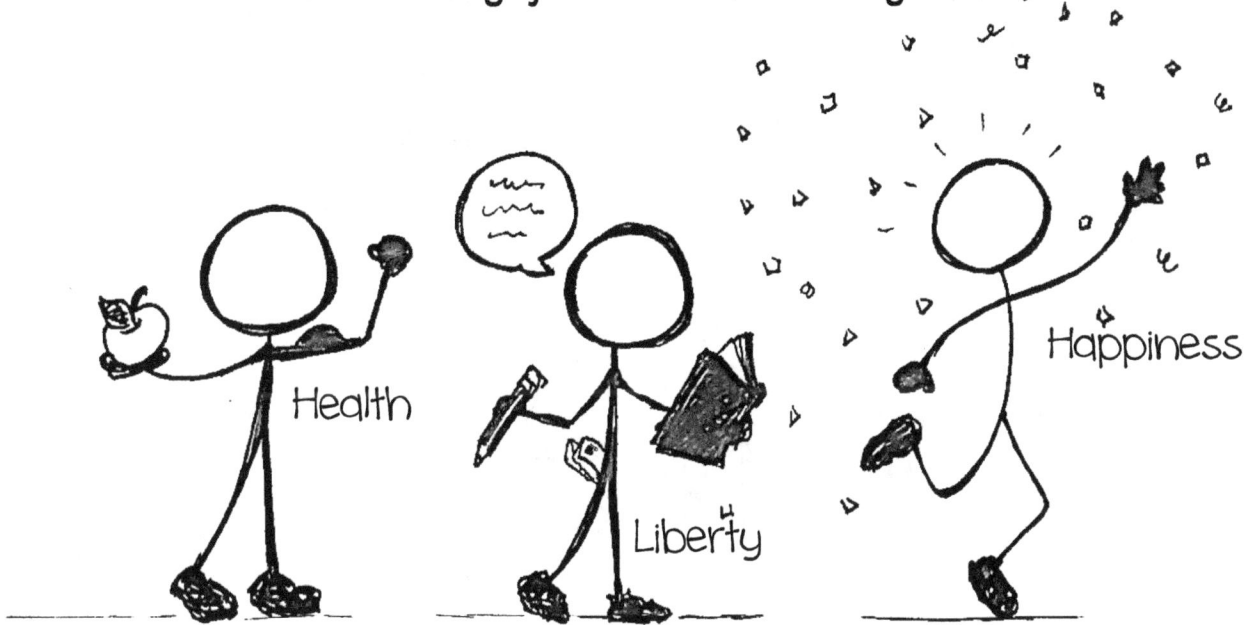

Health

Liberty

Happiness

_____

they want you to have a life filled with:
health, liberty, and happiness.

Yep, as strange as it seems,
it all comes down to these three things,
and embracing them is like giving you
and your whole generation wings!!

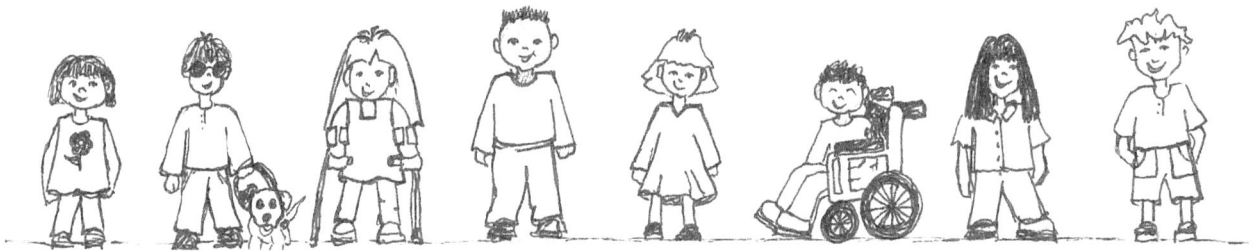

Sometimes grownups answer your questions with,
"Shhh, get it done, it is what's best for you."

This is just another way to say,
"It'll bring health and happiness,
with a life of liberty too!"

Health, liberty, and happiness are
extraordinary ideas and goals.

They can guide you as you reach your best,
while helping kids get along as a whole.

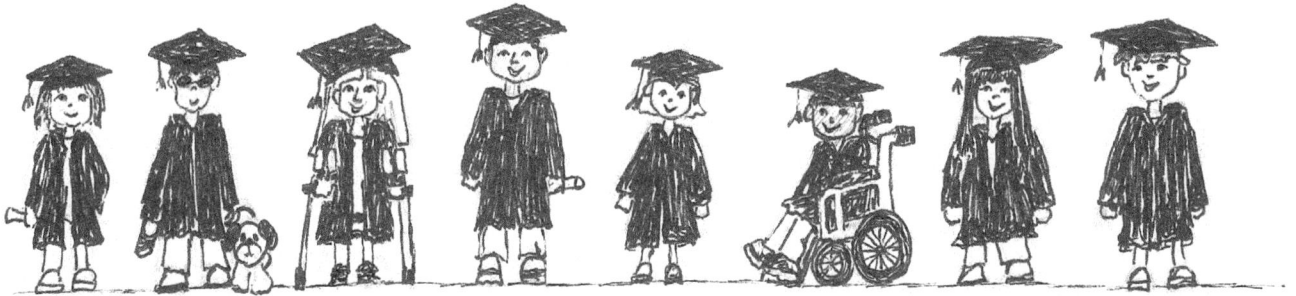

When you learn this truth,
and practice it too,

The three become great guidelines
for each day through.

Health, liberty, and happiness
are indeed a mouthful to say.
Some other goals can help groups thrive,
but you'll see, they're just not the same.

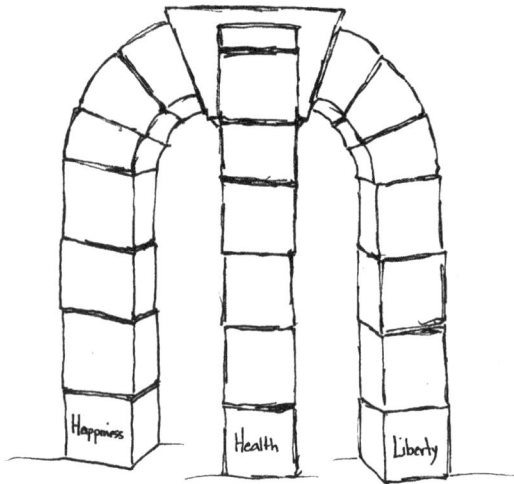

Like foundation stones
that are a building's solid
start,

these great ideas can be rules,
that let kids be safe while
they also follow their hearts!!

You see, these days many kids reach high
in schools of learning and togetherness!
But it used to be only a few could pursue
their health, liberty, and happiness.

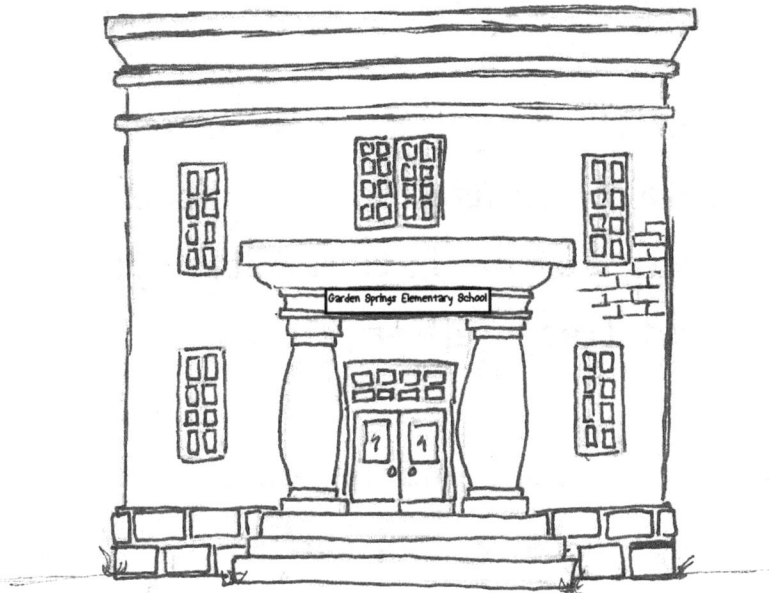

Yes, a long time ago, all over the world,
of these goals most people did not know.

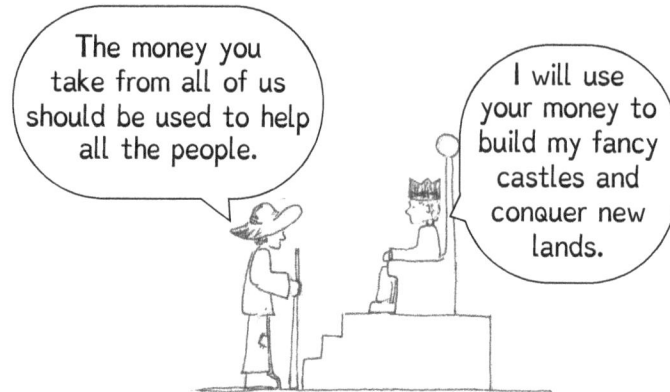

See, for thousands of years cruel leaders
unfairly controlled their people...
but we now have a better plan
that treats all people as equals.

Yes, before there were phones, cars, or airplane wings,
this world had many bossy, selfish queens and kings.
Sadly, they just took of their people's food,
land, money, and precious things.

The people got fed up and fought to have a say.
They dreamed of health and happiness,
and to be free in their own way.

We sure did need a simple plan,
one message all could use,
so we could stop wasting time,
and heal our humanity's blues.

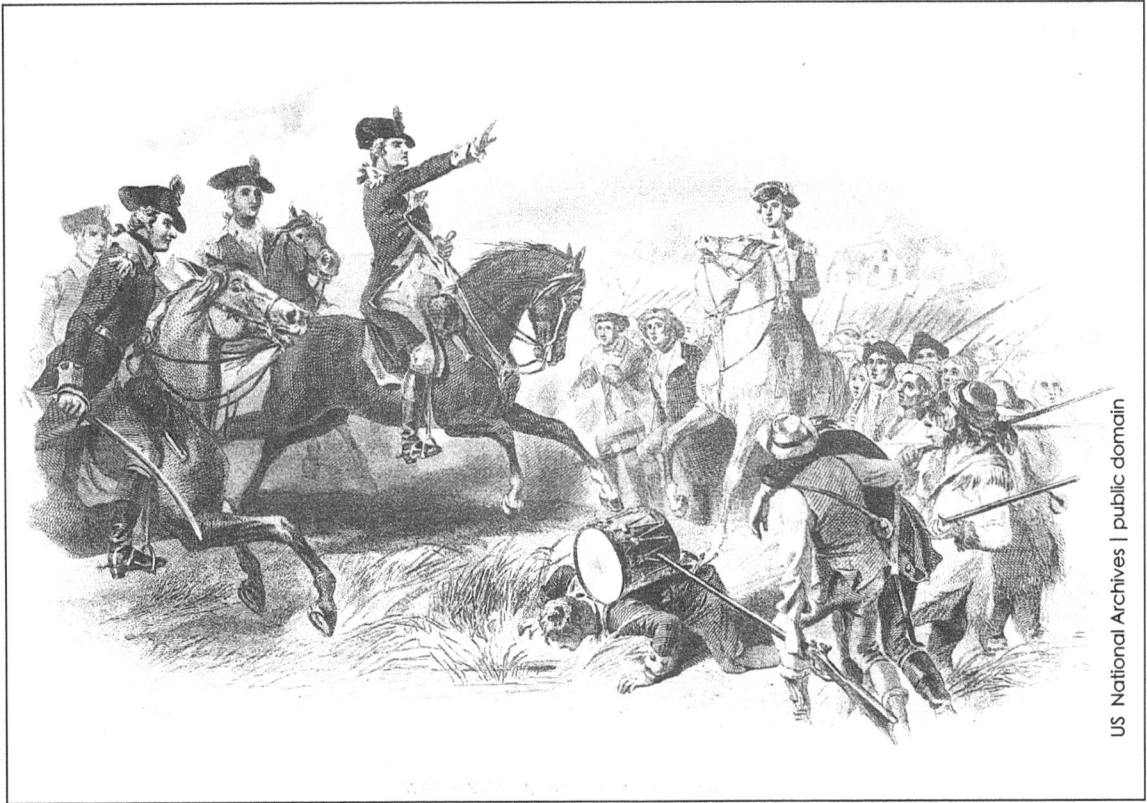

People starting thinking
and wrote these goals
into new rules and laws.

When we won the chance to
use them,
there was tremendous cheer
and applause!!

It was a new beginning for
the problems that needed
a big fix.
It was the year 1776!

We still have problems to fix but at least we are on track to a better future when all are considered equal.

IN CONGRESS. JULY 4, 1776.

The unanimous Declaration of the thirteen united States of America.

Underground Railroad

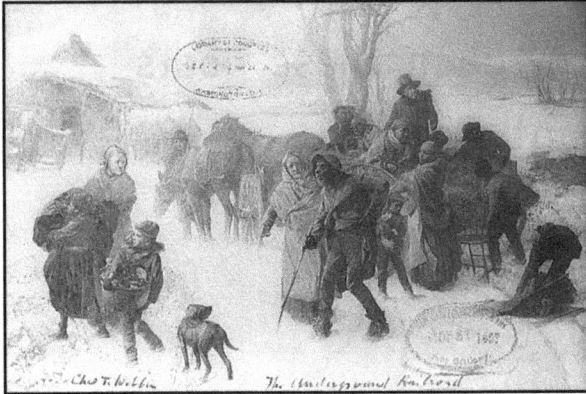

Abraham Lincoln | Union | Civil War

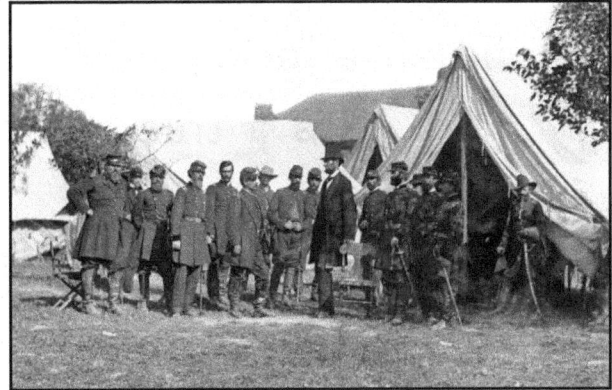

Normandy | WWII

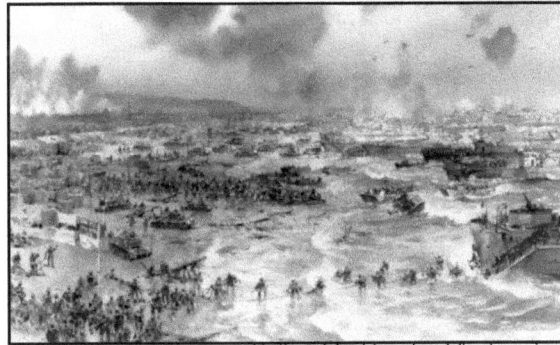

Yes, on these ideas and goals
people have thought, written, and fought,
and will continue to for years.
If we keep trying and keep holding them dear,
then surely to goodness they won't disappear.

We earthlings sure do need all the help we can get,
because losing the chance to reach these goals
is a true and constant threat.

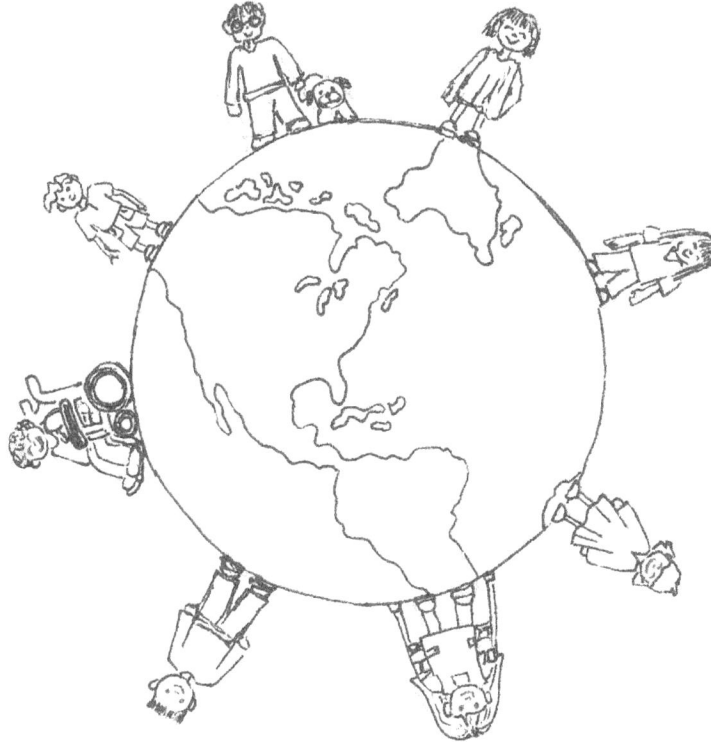

So you see,
you are all so very needed
in this many hundred year plan,
to make life fair
for every girl, boy, woman, and man.

Think and plan well....which job will you choose,
will you own a restaurant that serves barbecue?

Will you be a teacher, a doctor, storeowner, or mayor?
Perhaps a farmer, construction worker, or even a ball player?

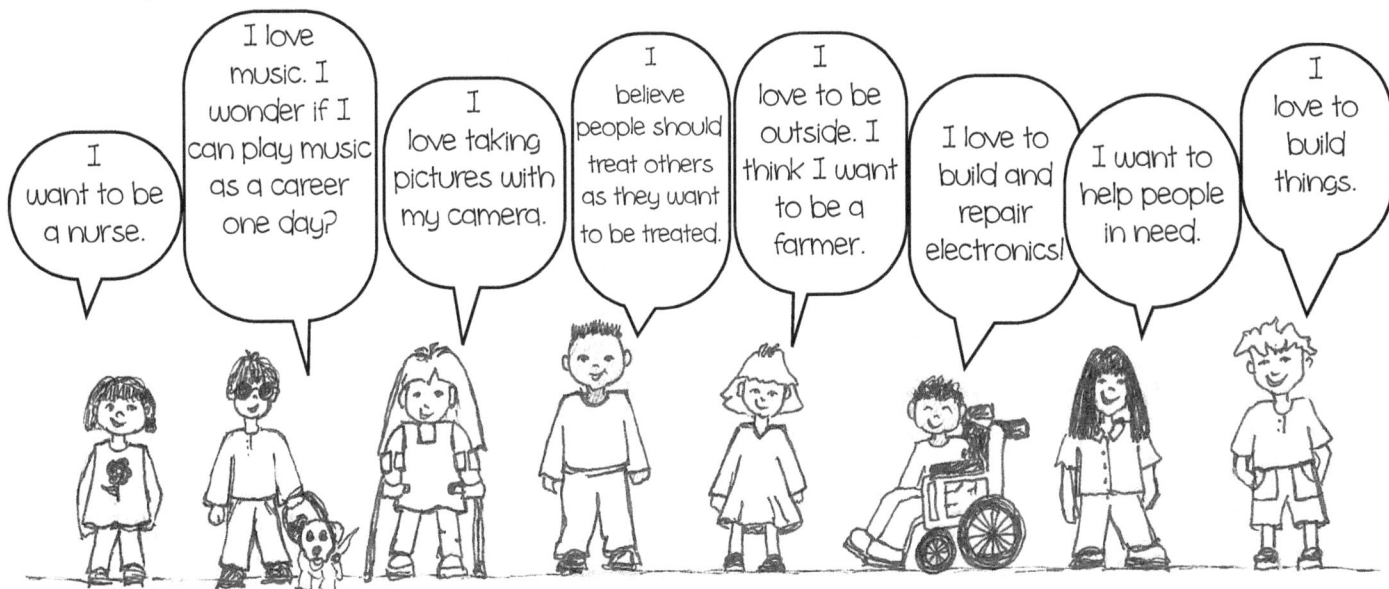

Maybe a pharmacist, a florist,
or a kind foster-mother?
What will you do to make our world better
for you and for others?
It's good to start thinking and dreaming of this now...
try all kinds of fun jobs, like milking a cow!

You see it's a privilege to reach for these goals,
because still many kids
don't get'a chance, you know!
You can even choose to see it as fun,
instead of being stressed as you go.

It's your good choices that help you
reach your potential,
in health, happiness, and liberty.

Like filling a cup to the top,
potential means fullest,
whether it's milk or ice tea.

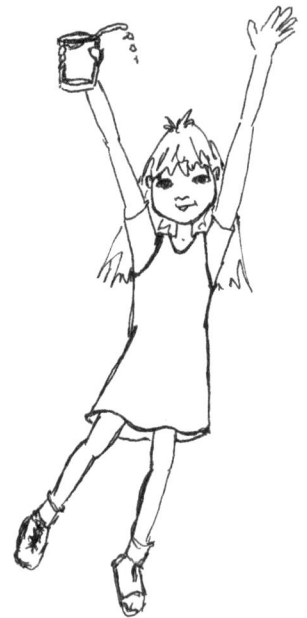

Just the same, your life can be filled up to the top
with great things of many kinds.
Your good choices, with help from grownups,
will build a great frame of mind!

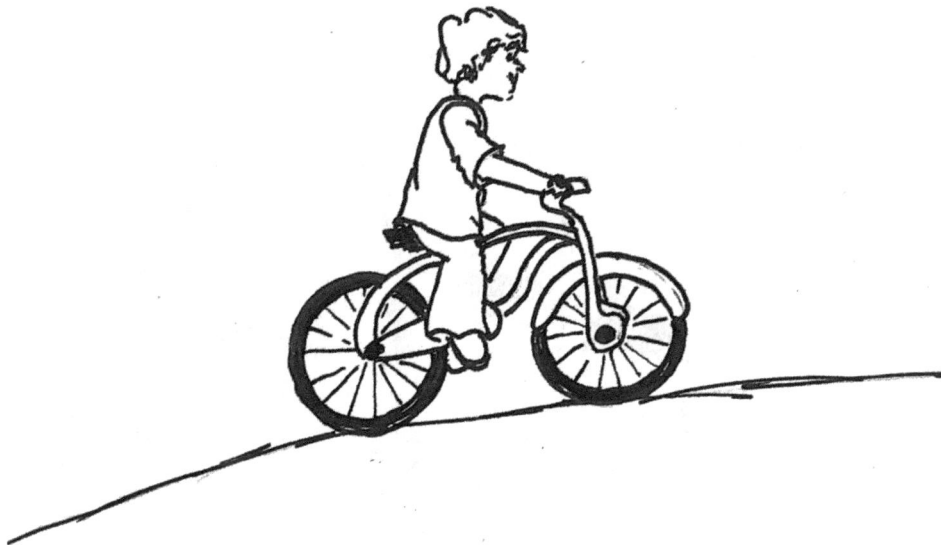

Now add the goal that we are also working together
for liberty, happiness, and health,
then we have a foundation for us all,
it's like building a common wealth!

It's also good to remember the grownups
who work hard for you each day,
See, they were kids once too
who had grownups helping *them* along the way.

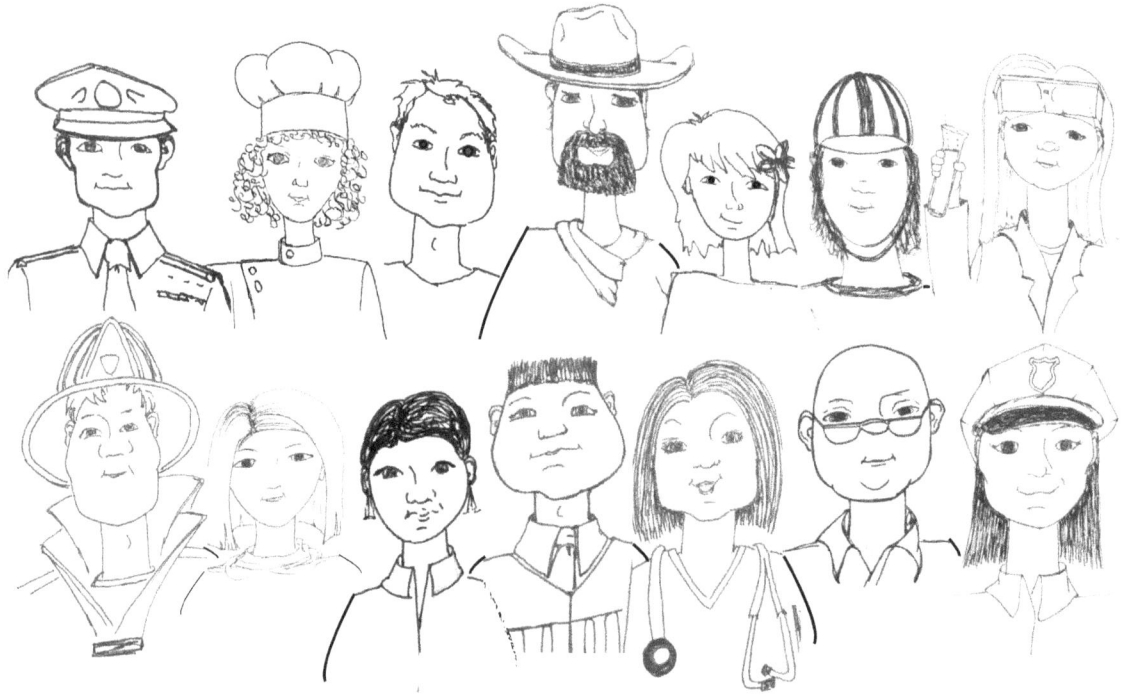

There are doctors, nurses, teachers, police,
and even your school's secretary...
scientists, bus drivers, farmers, vets,
and people who grow blueberries!

You see, its not just your family
who wants the best for you.

There are many people you've never met
who make the world better, it's true.

The world is better than ever before,
but there's still much work to do.

We need your generation's help
to make these goals possible for all kids to pursue.

More than ever before
your generation must work together,
we only have one blue green earth,
so your efforts must be clever.

Try your best, take care of yourself,
and at school do your best each minute.
Help other kids find a niche they love too,
or at least do not prevent it.

Good teamwork makes life sweeter,
just like honey from bees.
With mutual goals like these,
we can build a great school culture and society!

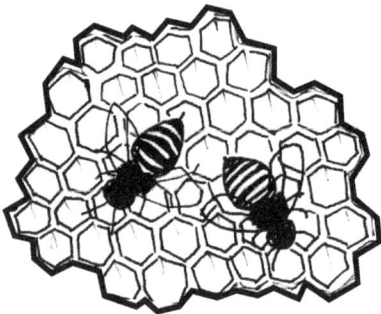

They can bring good order too
and prevent crazy commotion.
It's really quite simple
to put them into motion.

School Rules:

Health

1. Be organized and prepared.
2. Observe with all your senses.
3. Believe you can learn.
4. Be safe.

Liberty

5. Concentrate on your work.
6. Gain and practice skills.
7. Be purposeful with your goals.

Happiness

8. Be kind to others.
9. Do not prevent others from finding their niche.
10. Search for what brings you and friends happiness.
11. Graduate from high school find a way to take care of yourself and maybe others too!

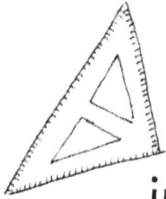

Say for example when you're in your class,
on the playground, or school bus,
just focus on reaching your own unique goals
of liberty, health, and happiness.

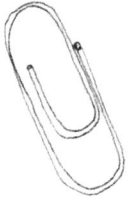

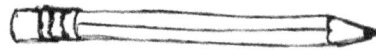

Remember,
fellow students
are doing the same
as they must,
keep in mind,
that your attitude
you might need to adjust.
Little by little you can find balance,
and build a world
of more respect and trust.

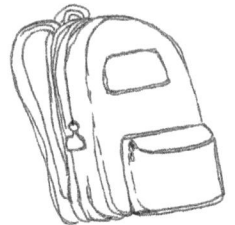

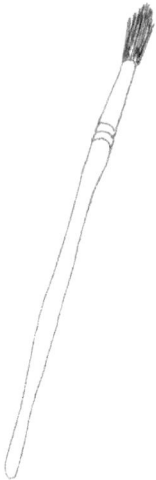

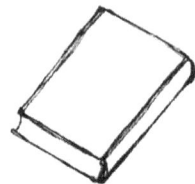

Teachers and parents will help with these goals,
all along the way.
If you need them, speak up, they can sort things out,
and help you know what to do and say.

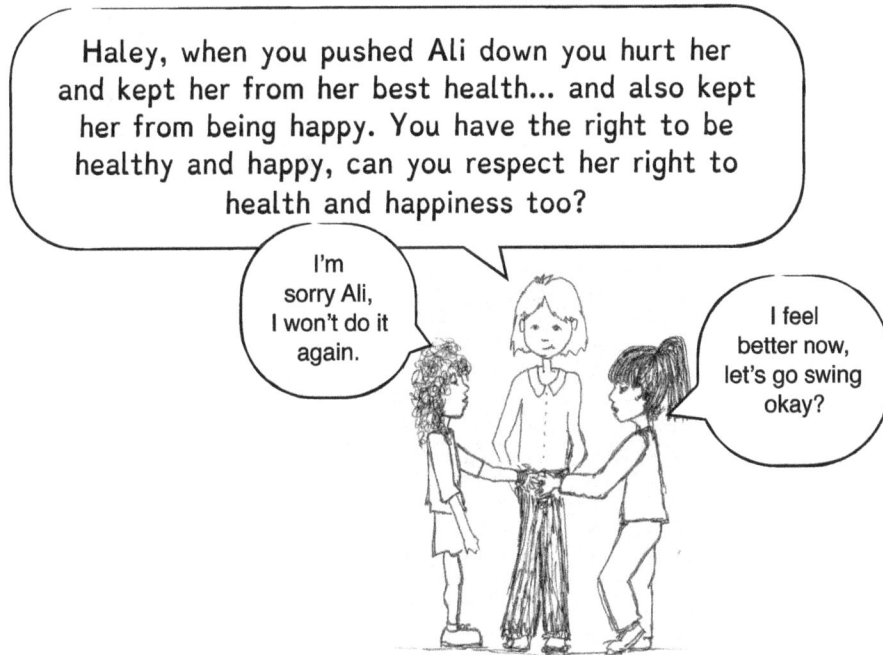

Haley, when you pushed Ali down you hurt her
and kept her from her best health... and also kept
her from being happy. You have the right to be
healthy and happy, can you respect her right to
health and happiness too?

I'm
sorry Ali,
I won't do it
again.

I feel
better now,
let's go swing
okay?

For example, out of the blue,
say a friend pushes you with a mean attitude,
If you tell them to stop and they keep on and on,
it's sure time to find a grownup and say,
"Please help me, c'mon!"

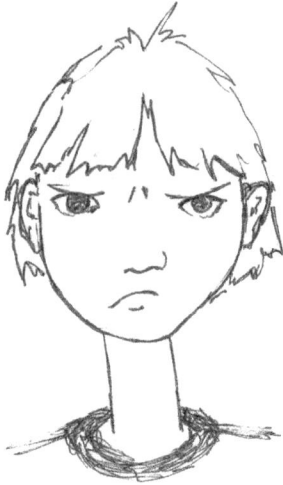

You must get help even
if the friend says,
"You are being a tattle tale,"
Sometimes kids just say that
so they can keep
leaving their mean attitude-trail.

What if they were mean to your friends,
your sister, or brother?
Better to fix things when you're young,
and learn to get along with one another.

Bullying keeps you from reaching your best,
tell a grownup and so you can stay on the road
to health, liberty, and happiness.

Sometimes kids don't mean to be bullies,
they just like to joke around,
it can be hard to tell,
be resilient, keep smiling,
don't let them make you frown.

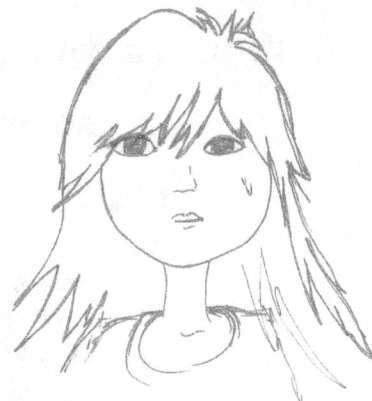

See, kids come from all kinds of families,
no two homes are alike.
Some families tease and goof a lot,
it's all in what they like.

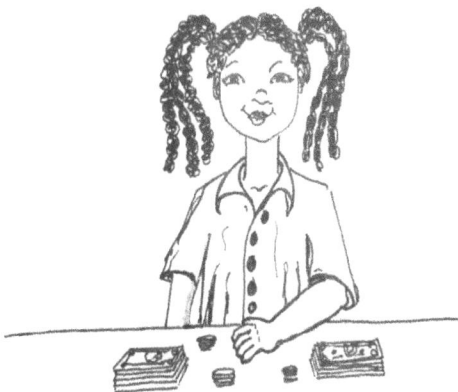

Remember, grownups bridge the gap,
and solve conflicts that arise.
All kids should feel good
about being at school,
there's always a compromise.

You are the one most in charge of your future days,
so make good choices, ask for help
and more great things will come your way.

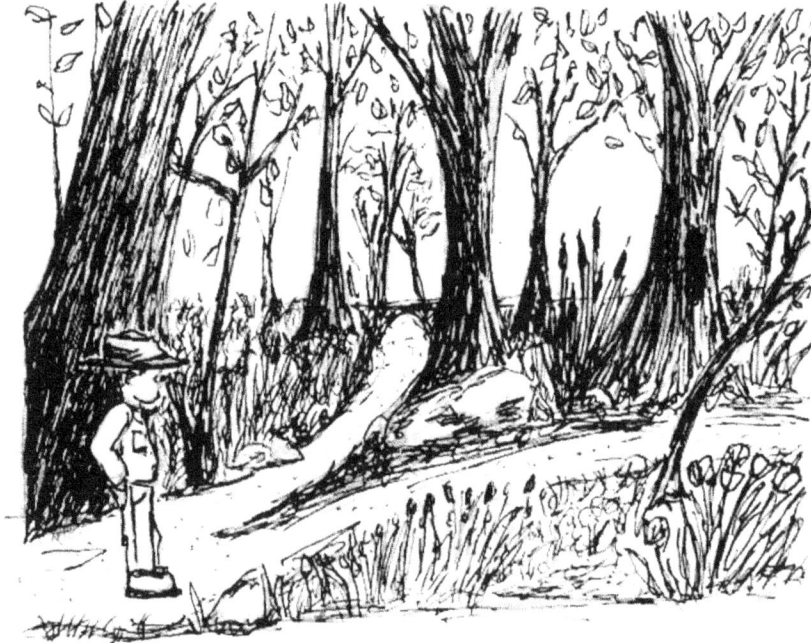

Like different paths along a trail,
ponder the best to take.
It's not so hard, as some might say,
Ask for help and follow through
with good choices that you make.

Some kids don't try their best on purpose,
it's hard to believe.
There's important work to do,
if we all do our best there's much we can achieve!

We've gotta find good fixes
so more people are happy, fed, and warm.
You see we don't have time to waste,
on choices that cause harm.

We earthlings have come
a long, long way,
but there are problems still to fix....
cures for diseases, solutions for hunger,
and answers to world conflicts.

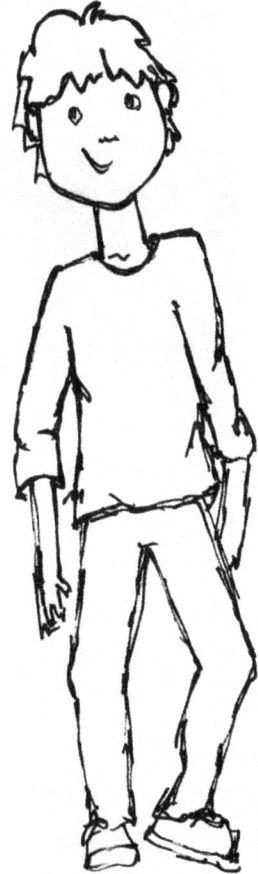

Helen Keller improved our world,
with just three senses: smell, taste, and touch.
She said, "Alone we can do so little,
together we can do so much."

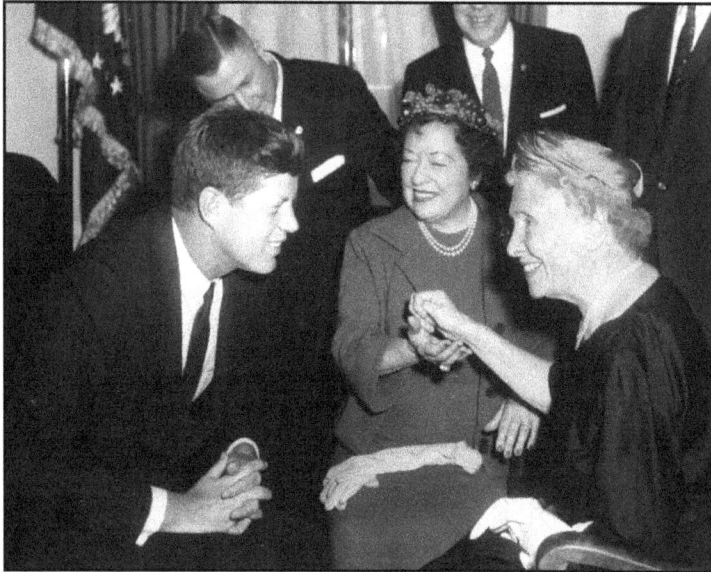

Helen Keller (right) was both blind and deaf from childhood. Her teacher, Annie Sullivan (center), taught her to "hear" and "speak" by using her hands to make specific shapes for different letters and words. Even though she lived in constant darkness and silence, she grew up to inspire thousands of people around the world with her positive, hopeful ideas. She even became friends with many leaders including the President of the United States, John F. Kennedy (left).

photo: Abby Rowe | JFK Library | public domain

No matter your station, learning level, or race,
there's a job and a life that is your just-right place.

So, keep searching and dreaming and trying your best,
to seek your potential of
health, liberty, and happiness!

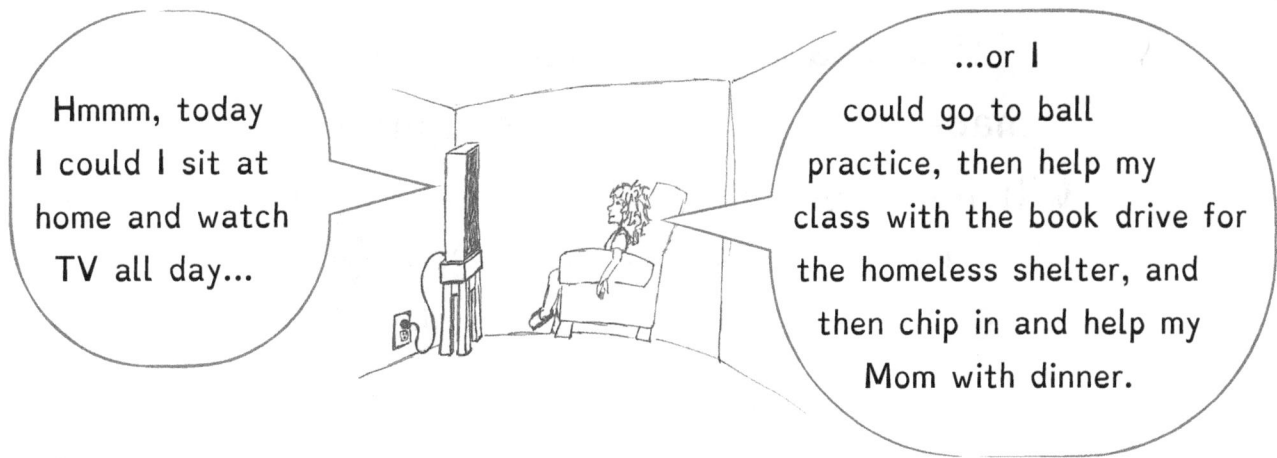

Hmmm, today I could I sit at home and watch TV all day...

...or I could go to ball practice, then help my class with the book drive for the homeless shelter, and then chip in and help my Mom with dinner.

Again, there's no reason to feel stressed,
for this work can be such fun,
and, hey, some of this work you've already done!

Yes, you've learned to get dressed
and eat all by yourself.
I bet you can read several books that sit on your shelf!

These things are easy now, but were difficult at first.
Simply keep learning, working, playing, resting...
and have nutritious food interspersed!

It's amazing how good choices,
made while you're young right now,
will help you when you're all grown up,
to get a job or buy a house.

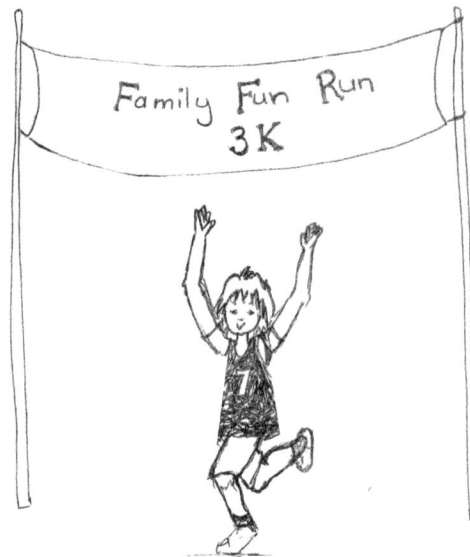

So set fun goals,
and practice hard along the way.
Like, you could run a little each day,
until you finish an entire 3k!

Now, everyone makes mistakes sometimes,
even grownups get frustrated!
Never give up on the right path,
and on good choices stay concentrated.

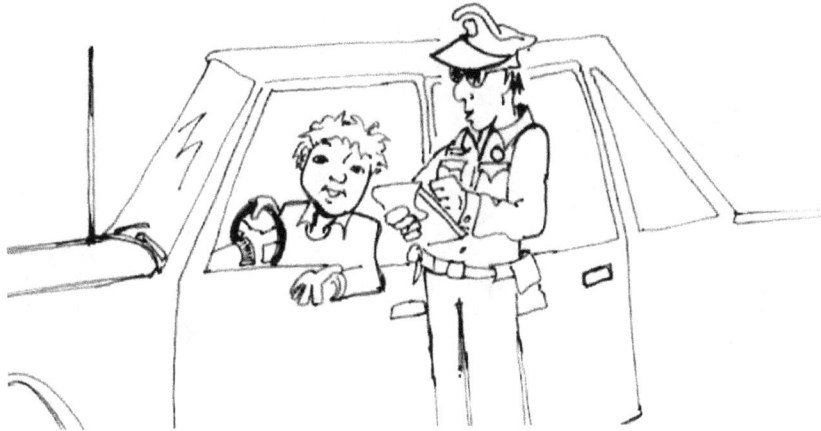

Wrong choices can even teach you,
the next time you'll try something different, it's true.
The better you get at making good choices,
the more great things can happen for you!

To sum it up, it's good to see our goals
as fair and excellent.
It's why the huddled masses still come
as hopeful immigrants.

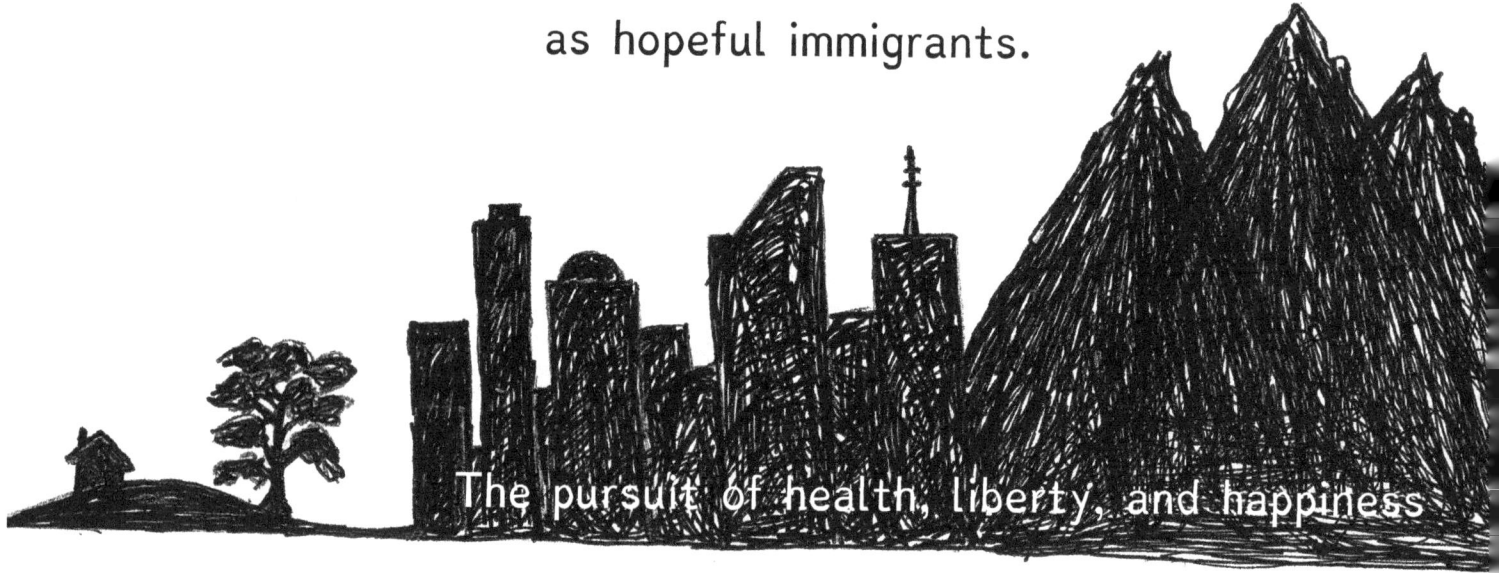

The pursuit of health, liberty, and happiness

Yes, each country has different goals
that work best for them, it's true.
We can respect theirs as we value and keep ours too!

Families also have different customs and beliefs,
if we strive for our three goals,
we will reach more concord and relief.

You see from long ago until today
we humans have struggled so,
to get along, be well, and make enough food grow.

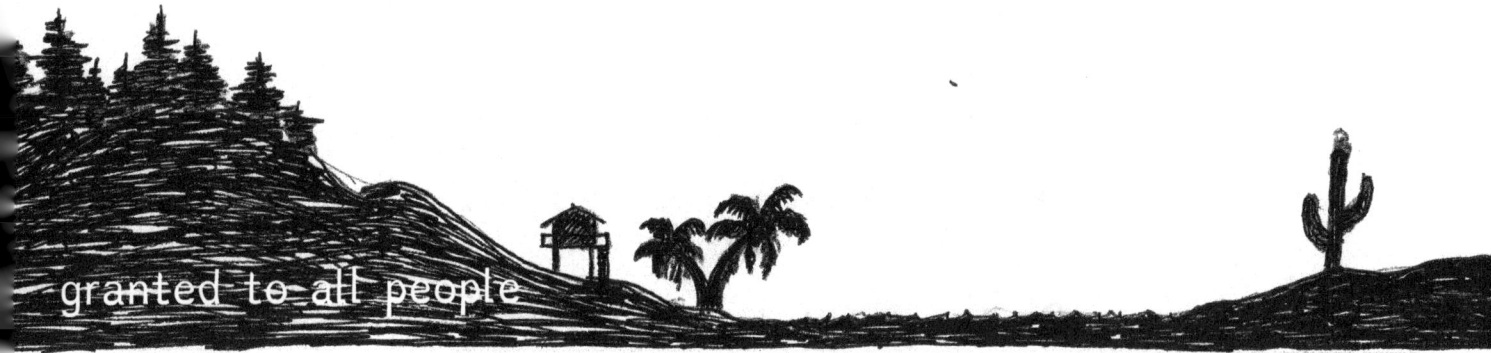

granted to all people

With all our different backgrounds and many colors of skin,
we still just need a simple plan
toward a solution we can believe in.

So remember, respect other ideas
that bring color to our world,
while preserving our three goals that bring
bright futures for boys and girls.

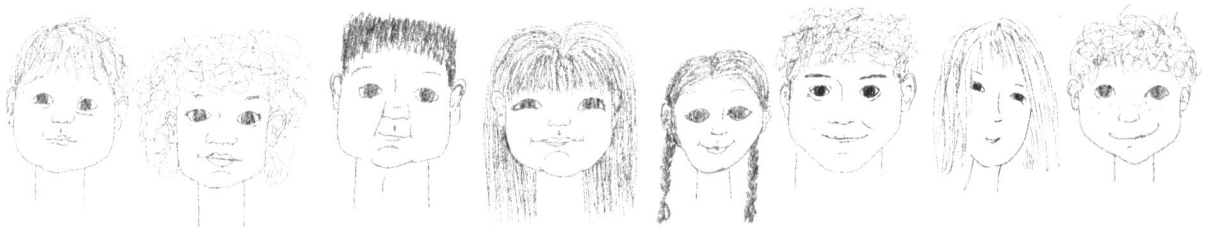

All this rhyming is a little silly,
yes, we know,
we hope you now grasp why
grownups ask so much as you grow!

So laugh a lot, keep making plans,
and be sure to check on the weather.
And always try your best
to eat good meals together.

Sing songs with friends
and exercise often in a week's time.
And remember read books like this one...
that rhyme!

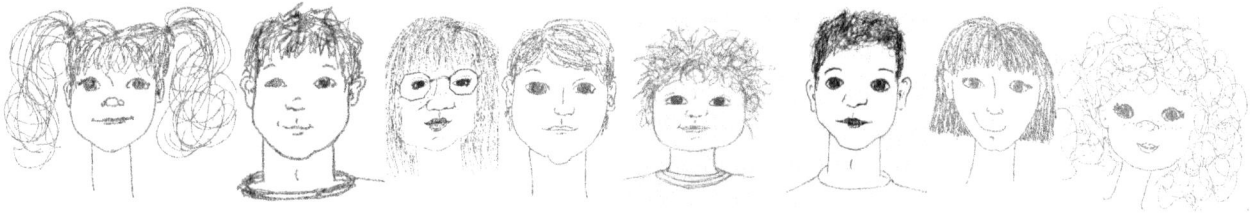

Finish your pages of math problems,
and your words correctly spell.
Always try your best and
listen to your lessons well.

Don't forget to brush your teeth,
and wash your smiley face.
Be on time for school each day,
for you are indeed a needed part of our human race!

We grownups wish for you and your whole generation
great friendship and success....
for we all hope you each reach your potential
of health, liberty, and true happiness!!

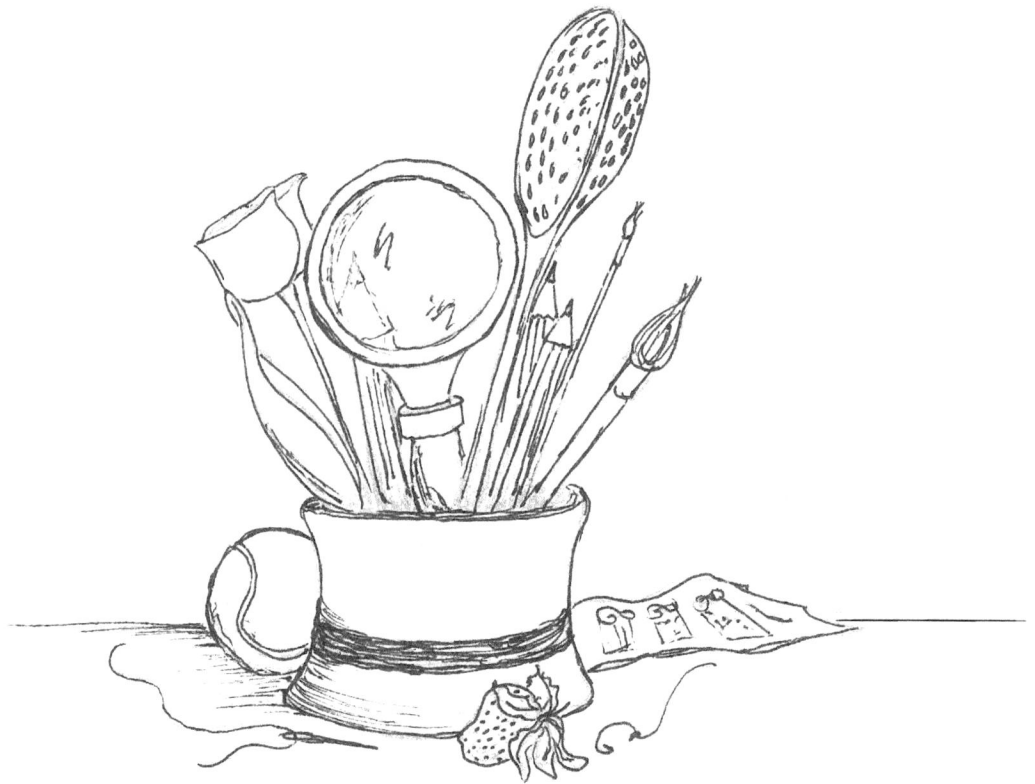

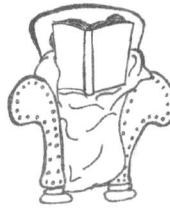

The book
Why Do Grownups Ask Us to Do So Much?
and other books written
by Stephanie Fairchild Fister
can be found on Amazon.com and Whatsbestforourkids.com

Journal Pages:

How will you reach your potential
of health, liberty, and happiness?

This book is a place to keep a list
of your choices toward success.

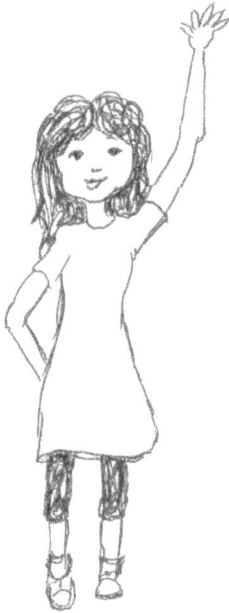

Simply write down your memories,
goals, and activities on the following
pages,

there's room for photos and report
cards too
for each of your school-age stages!

You can then share this book
with your teachers every year.
They care how you learn best,
so you can get the most out of your school career!

This book can be a record and a place for memories too,
where you can look back and see one day,
the first years of you!!

You were born on

_____

Key things to remember about your first year (birth to 1)

Things to include on this page:

Did someone read books aloud to you everyday? What were your favorites? Did you get to sing and listen to music everyday? What were your favorite songs? Did you get to go outside most everyday?

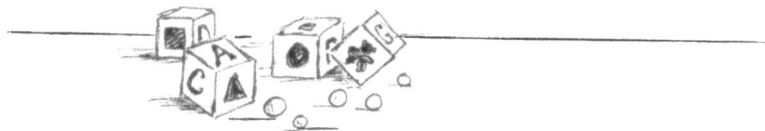

Things to remember from when you were one year old:

(One to Two years old)

Things to include on this page:

Did someone read books aloud to you everyday? What were your favorites? Did you get to sing and listen to music everyday? What were your favorites? Did you get to go outside most everyday?

Important things to remember about when you were two years old:

Did someone read books aloud to you everyday? What were your favorites? Did you get to sing and listen to music everyday? What were your favorites? Did you get to play outside most everyday? What did you love to do? Did you learn to wash your hands and eat all by yourself?

Three years old:

Did someone read books aloud to you everyday? What were your favorites? Did you get to sing and listen to music everyday? What were your favorite songs? Did you recognize any letters or words when you were three? Did you get to play outside most everyday? What did you love to do? Did you participate in any classes or sports? Who were your favorite friends when you were three?

Four years old:

Did someone read books aloud to you everyday? What were your favorites? Did you get to sing and listen to music everyday? What were your favorite songs? Did you recognize any letters or words when you were four? Did you get to play outside most everyday? What did you love to do? Did you participate in any classes or sports? Who were your favorite friends when you were four?

Five years old:

Did someone read books aloud to you everyday? What were your favorites? Did you get to sing and listen to music everyday? What were your favorite songs? Did you recognize any letters or words when you were five? Did you get to play outside most everyday? What did you love to do? Did you participate in any classes or sports? Who were your favorite friends when you were five?

Six years old:

Did someone read books aloud to you everyday? What were your favorites? Did you get to sing and listen to music everyday? What were your favorite songs? Did you read any books by yourself? Did you get to play outside most everyday? What did you love to do? What classes or sports did you participate in? Who were your favorite friends when you were six?

Seven years old:

Did someone read books aloud to you everyday? What were your favorites? Did you get to sing and listen to music everyday? What were your favorite songs? Did you read any books? Did you get to play outside most everyday? What did you love to do? What classes or sports did you participate in? Who were your favorite friends?

Eight years old:

Did someone read books aloud to you everyday? What were your favorites? Did you get to sing and listen to music everyday? What were your favorite songs? Did you read any books? Did you get to play outside most everyday? What did you love to do? What classes or sports did you participate in? Who were your favorite friends?

Nine years old:

Did someone read books aloud to you everyday? What were your favorites? Did you get to sing and listen to music everyday? What were your favorite songs? Did you read any books? Did you get to play outside most everyday? What did you love to do? What classes or sports did you participate in? Who were your favorite friends?

Ten years old:

Did someone read books aloud to you everyday? What were your favorites? Did you get to sing and listen to music everyday? What were your favorite songs? Did you read any books? Did you get to play outside most everyday? What did you love to do? What classes or sports did you participate in? Who were your favorite friends?

Eleven years old:

Did someone read books aloud to you everyday? What were your favorites? Did you get to sing and listen to music everyday? What were your favorite songs? Did you read any books? Did you get to play outside most everyday? What did you love to do? What classes or sports did you participate in? Who were your favorite friends?

Twelve years old:

Did someone read books aloud to you everyday? What were your favorites? Did you get to sing and listen to music everyday? What were your favorite songs? Did you read any books? Did you get to play outside most everyday? What did you love to do? What classes or sports did you participate in? Who were your favorite friends?

www.ingramcontent.com/pod-product-compliance
Lightning Source LLC
Chambersburg PA
CBHW080148310326
41914CB00090B/897

*9 7 8 0 9 7 4 0 0 6 4 0 6 *